I0417381

APPLE SMOOTHIE

2 c Apple sauce

1 c Apple cider

1 c Orange juice

2 tb Vermont maple syrup

1/2 ts Nutmeg

1/2 ts Cinnamon

Combine all ingredients in a blender and blend until smooth. Pour into glasses and serve. Serves 2.

APPLE APRICOT SMOOTHIE

1 Golden Delicious apple, peeled, cored and chopped
1 c apple juice
4 apricots, fresh, pitted -skin optional
1 banana; peeled
3/4 c plain or vanilla nonfat yogurt
10 ice cubes, up to 12 cubes
1 Tbsp. honey

Place all ingredients in a blender and puree until smooth.

APPLE BANANA SOY SMOOTHIE

2 ripe bananas, peeled and halved
2 apples, peeled, cored and quartered
300ml (10fl oz) nonfat yogurt
2 tbsp sugar
400ml (15fl oz) organic soya milk

Put all the ingredients in a blender and purée for 1 minute.

APPLE BERRY SMOOTHIE

½ cup O.J.
1 Cup fresh Apple Cider
4-6 Strawberries with stem left on

1 Frozen Banana 1 cup Yogurt (Sugar & Fat Free flavored)
¼ cup Almonds
2 Tbs. Wheat Germ
Blend until a nice smooth consistency. This makes enough for 3.

APPLE CINNAMON SMOOTHIE

3/4 cup Apple Sugarfree Syrup

1/4 cup Cinnamon Sugarfree Syrup

2 scoops VegeFuel

1 1/2 cups crushed ice

1/4 cup Heavy Cream (optional)

Blend until smooth.

APPLE COCONUT SMOOTHIE

1/4 cup apple juice

1 pinch grated coconut or 1 T. coconut milk

1/2 banana

1/4 teaspoon fresh ginger root peeled

2 small ice cubes

Put all ingredients into blender.

Blend until smoothie consistency is reached!

APPLE COCONUT GINGER SMOOTHIE

1/4 c Apple juice

1 pn Coconut -- grated OR_ -1 Tbsp coconut milk

1/2 ea Banana

1/4 ts Ginger root -- fresh,peeled -grated

1/2 c -Crushed ice -- or 2 small ice -Cubes

Blend all until smooth.

APPLE MAPLE SMOOTHIE

2 c apple sauce
1 c apple cider
1 c orange juice
2 Tbsp. Vermont maple syrup
1/2 tsp. nutmeg
1/2 tsp. cinnamon

Combine all ingredients in a blender and blend until smooth. Pour into glasses and serve.

APPLE PIE A-LA-MODE SMOOTHIE

2 cup frozen vanilla yogurt, nonfat
3/4 cup unsweetened applesauce
1/4 cup apple juice, chilled
1 cup apple, peeled and diced
1/2 teaspoon cinnamon
1/4 teaspoon ground nutmeg

Combine the frozen yogurt, applesauce, and apple juice in a blender. Add the apple, cinnamon, and nutmeg. Blend until smooth.

APRICOT MANGO SMOOTHIE

6 oz. light (reduced sugar) fat-free Apricot-Mango yogurt

(This is one container of Yoplait)

1 cup. Crystal Light lemonade

1/2 banana

5-6 canned apricot halves

Put all ingredients into blender. Blend well until smoothie consistency is reached!

APRICOT NECTARINE SMOOTHIE

1/2 nectarine

1 apricot

6 oz. light (reduced sugar) fat-free peach yogurt, frozen

(This is one container of Yoplait)

4 oz. Crystal Light or other sugar-free lemonade

Put all ingredients into blender. Blend until smoothie consistency is reached!

APRICOT SMOOTHIE

1/4 cup orange juice
1/2 cup plain, low-fat yogurt
1/2 cup peeled, pitted and chopped fresh apricots
honey to taste
Place all the ingredients in a blender. Blend on high speed until smooth.

BAHAMA MAMA SMOOTHIE

1/4 cup tofu
1 1/2 cups tropical V-8 Splash or other pineapple/citrus blend
1/4 cup plain non fat yogurt
1/2 banana
Frozen strawberries, pineapple, and mango
water or soy milk to taste/consistency

Optional:
3 or 4 baby carrots (you'll never know they're in there!)
1 tbs. wheat germ or 4-5 almonds

Blend all ingredients in blender until smooth.

BANANA SMOOTHIE

1 banana
1 cup of plain yoghurt
1 cup of orange juice
Blend until smooth.

BANANA-APRICOT SHAKE

1 cup mashed ripe bananas -- (about 2 large), -- frozen

1/2 cup low-fat milk

1 cup apricot nectar

1/4 teaspoon vanilla

Place all ingredients in blender. Cover and blend about 30 seconds or until smooth. Serve immediately over ice cubes. Serves 2.

BANANA BERRY SMOOTHIE

2 bananas

1/2 cup blueberries

1 cup plain yogurt

Peel bananas, slice and place on a cookie sheet. Put in freezer and freeze until solid. Remove from freezer and place in blender. Slice berries and add to blender. Pour in yogurt. Blend until smooth. Pour into glass and serve.

BANANA-BERRY POWER SMOOTHIE

1/4 cup orange juice
1/2 cup plain, low-fat yogurt
1/2 small, peeled ripe banana
1/4 cup stemmed, sliced strawberries
honey to taste
1 1/2 tablespoons vanilla soy protein powder
Place all the ingredients in a blender. Blend on high speed until smooth.

BANANA CINNAMON SMOOTHIE

In a blender combine:
1/4 c plain yogurt (I actually use vanilla for mine but it would depend on what else you're adding)
1/4 c skim milk
1/2 banana
A splash of vanilla
A dash of cinnamon
4 ice cubes
Blend to desired consistency. Substitute whatever fruit is in season or even use something like canned peaches. I usually double the recipe above but this is what I remember the original measurements to be.

BANANA COFFEE SMOOTHIE

2 small bananas, peeled, cut up, and frozen
1 1/2 cups skim milk
1 8-oz. container low-fat coffee yogurt
1/4 tsp. ground cinnamon
Dash ground nutmeg

In a blender container combine frozen bananas, milk, yogurt, cinnamon, and nutmeg. Cover and blend till smooth. To serve, pour into glasses. If desired, garnish with fresh bananas and mint.

BANANA CREAMA SMOOTHIE

1 banana

½ cup natural yogurt
2 cups milk
2 teaspoons pure vanilla essence
Slice banana and put into a blender. Add ½ cup milk, yogurt and vanilla. Blend until banana is mushed. Add remaining milk and blend until smooth. Pour into glasses.

BANANA FRUIT SMOOTHIE

1 cup orange juice
2 cups plain low-fat yogurt
4 small bananas
honey to taste
Place all the ingredients in a blender. Blend on high speed until smooth.

BANANA LIME SUBLIME SMOOTHIE

2 cups limeade
1 banana
1 cup lime sherbet
3 Tbs. coconut milk
1 cup ice Pour all liquid ingredients into the blender. Add all frozen ingredients. Blend at MIX setting for 30 seconds then blend at SMOOTH setting until smooth. While the machine is running, move the stir stick around counter-clockwise to aid mixing. Serve immediately. Each recipe serves 3-5.

BANANA MOLASSES SMOOTHIE

5 pitted prunes
1 medium banana, peeled and cut into 1-inch pieces
2 cups low-fat vanilla soymilk.
1 tablespoon blackstrap molasses
1/4 teaspoon ground cardamom
3 ice cubes

Place prunes in small bowl and cover with hot tap water. Let rest for 15 minutes or until plump. Drain. Combine plumped prunes and remaining ingredients in blender and whip until smooth.

BANANA OAT SMOOTHIE

1 Cup Milk

1 Packet Instant Oatmeal, Regular Flavor

1 Whole Banana, Cut In Chunks

1 Cup Orange Juice

Combine all ingredients in a blender. Cover and blend on high speed for 1 min.

BANANA ORANGE SMOOTHIE

1 8-ounce container nonfat cherry yogurt
1 banana, peeled, cut into pieces
1 orange, peeled, white pith removed, cut into segments
8 frozen dark cherries
6 frozen strawberries

Combine ingredients in blender. Blend on medium speed until smooth. Divide between 2 glasses.

BANANA PEACH SMOOTHIE

1 cup mashed ripe bananas -- (about 2 large), -- frozen

1 cup peach nectar

1/2 cup low-fat milk

Place all ingredients in blender. Cover and blend about 30 seconds or until smooth. Serve immediately over ice cubes. Serves 2.

BANANA PEANUT BUTTER SMOOTHIE

8 oz skim milk
1/3 small banana
1 tbsp reduced fat peanut butter
2 sweet n' low or other sugar substitute
5 ice cubes

In blender combine milk, banana, peanut butter and sweet n' low. Add ice cubes and pulse.

BANANA PINEAPPLE COLADA SMOOTHIE

1/2 peeled banana
1/2 cup pineapple chunks
1/2 cup pineapple juice
1/2 cup ice cubes
1 tablespoon sugar
1/4 teaspoon coconut extract

Place all ingredients in a blender and blender until smooth.

BANANA SOY SMOOTHIE

3/4 cup soy milk
1/2 cup soft silken tofu
4 bananas, frozen
1 tablespoon honey
1 tablespoon vanilla extract

1 tablespoon carob powder

Combine soy milk and tofu in blender. Add bananas, honey, vanilla extract, and carob powder. Blend until smooth.

BANANA SPICE SMOOTHIE

1 ripe banana, chopped
2 tablespoons low fat natural yogurt 1-2 teaspoons honey (to taste)
180ml cold milk (low fat or soy may be used)
Nutmeg
Place all ingredients, except nutmeg, into a blender and blend until smooth. Pour into a tall glass, sprinkle with nutmeg if desired and serve immediately. For a delicious nutty taste, try adding 1 tablespoon of slivered almonds to the blender.

BANANA STRAWBERRY ORANGE

1 banana
1 handful of strawberries
1 cup vanilla yogurt
1/2 cup milk
1/2 cup orange juice
a handful of ice cubes
Put it all in the blender. Serves 3.

BANANALICIOUS SMOOTHIE

1 cup orange juice
2 cups plain low-fat yogurt
4 small bananas
honey to taste
Peel the bananas and measure the orange juice and yogurt. Place all the ingredients in a blender. Blend on low speed until smooth.

BEAM ME UP BANANA SMOOTHIE

2 bananas (frozen)

1 cup of strawberries

1 cup of vanilla rice milk

2 cap full of Vanilla Extract

4 tablespoons of Grade B Maple Syrup

1/10 teaspoon of nutmeg

Place all ingredients in blender, mix and drink

BERRY SMOOTHIE

I small container (6 oz) nonfat yogurt (any flavor)
1 cup skim milk
1 cup frozen berries (any type)

Blend on high till smooth. You could add a few chunks of banana if you prefer. Serves 1.

BERRY BANANA SMOOTHIE

1 small banana, peeled, cut up, and frozen
1/4 cup fresh or frozen assorted berries (such as strawberries, blackberries, and/or raspberries)
1 cup orange juice
3 tablespoons low-fat vanilla yogurt
Sliced fresh strawberries (optional)
In a blender container combine the frozen banana pieces, desired berries, orange juice, and yogurt. Cover and blend till smooth. To serve, pour into tall glasses. If desired, garnish each drink with fresh strawberries.

BERRY BLAST SMOOTHIE

1 cup apple juice
1 1/2 cups lemonade
1 cup frozen raspberries
1/2 cup frozen strawberries
1 cup raspberry sherbet Pour all liquid ingredients into the blender. Add all frozen ingredients. Blend at MIX setting for 30 seconds then blend at SMOOTH setting until smooth. While the machine is running, move the stir stick around counter-clockwise to aid mixing. Serve immediately. Each recipe serves 3-5.

BERRY BRAINSTORM SMOOTHIE

1/2 cup frozen strawberries
1/2 cup frozen blueberries
1/2 cup frozen raspberries
1/2 cup apple juice
1/2 tsp. lemon juice
1/2 cup nonfat frozen yogurt
1/2 cup ice

Combine ingredients in blender; mix until smooth and frothy. Serves 1.

BERRY DELICIOUS SMOOTHIE

1/4 cup orange juice
1/2 cup plain, low-fat yogurt
1/6 cup washed, stemmed raspberries
1/6 cup washed, stemmed blackberries
1/6 cup washed, stemmed blueberries
honey to taste
Wash berries and remove stems. Place all the ingredients in a blender. Blend on high speed until smooth.

BERRY GOOD PEACH SMOOTHIE

1/2 cup apple juice
1/2 cup nonfat vanilla yogurt
1 cup fresh peaches, sliced, partially frozen
1/2 cup raspberries, partially frozen
1 1/2 cups ice chips

Pour ingredients into a blender and blend until smooth. Serves 2.

BLACK AND BLUE SMOOTHIE

1/4 cup blueberries

1/4 cup blackberries

1 banana

1/2 cup apple juice

1/3 cup raspberry sorbet

Put all ingredients into blender.

Blend until smoothie consistency is reached!

BLACK CHERRY SMOOTHIE

5 huge tablespoons of yoghurt
0.5 cup of frozen black cherries
sweeten with honey
Blend until smooth.

BLUEBERRY SMOOTHIE

1 cup frozen blueberries

8 oz fat free yogurt

milk to thin (Skim is fine)

Process in blender. Because the berries are frozen, the result is almost like a malt. If I use plain yogurt, I add a little sugar or Equal and sometimes vanilla. Or, I have used blueberry or lemon yogurt. Makes 2 servings.

BLUEBERRY BANANA SMOOTHIE

1 ripe medium banana
3/4 cup fresh or frozen blueberries
1/4 cup nonfat vanilla yogurt
3/4 cup skim milk
pinch of cinnamon (if desired)
1/2 cup of crushed ice

Combine all of the ingredients in a blender and puree until smooth. Serves 2

BLUEBERRY BLAST SMOOTHIE

1/2 frozen bannana (or unfrozen + 1 ice cube)

1/4-1/2 c frozen blueberries

1/2-3/4 c rice dream vanilla lite

1/2 tsp vanilla extract

1 pkt sweetner (I use sweet one)

Dump it all in the blender and whir until creamy.

BLUEBERRY BUTTERMILK SMOOTHIE

1 banana, ripe, peeled and cut into chunks
1/2 cup frozen blueberries
1 tablespoon granulated sugar
4 ice cubes
1 cup buttermilk

Place all ingredients in blender and process until smooth. Serves 2

BLUEBERRY PINEAPPLE SMOOTHIE

2 cups chilled fresh or frozen blueberries, slightly thawed
1 cup chilled pineapple-orange juice, or pineapple-orange-strawberry juice
1 8-ounce carton vanilla nonfat yogurt
1 tablespoon sugar

In a blender container, combine all ingredients. Cover and blend for 1 to 2 minutes or until almost smooth. Makes 3 servings.

BLUEBERRY SMOOTHIE

1/4 cup orange juice
1/2 cup plain, low-fat yogurt
1/2 cup washed, stemmed blueberries
honey to taste
Place all the ingredients in a blender. Blend on high speed until smooth.

BLUEBERRY TWIST SMOOTHIE

2 cups fresh blueberries
1 cup pineapple orange juice
1- 8 ounce vanilla yogurt
2 teaspoons sugar or honey

Place everything in a blender. Blend until SMOOTH! Serve immediately. Serves 2.

BOYSENBERRY BLUEBERRY SMOOTHIE

1 1/2 cups boysenberry or blackberry-flavor juice
1 cup boysenberries or blackberries
1 cup blueberries, frozen

Place all ingredients in blender and process until smooth. Serves 2

BREAKFAST SMOOTHIE

1/2 cup orange juice

1 banana

6-7 frozen strawberries

4-5 slices frozen peaches

5-6 frozen blueberries

6-7 ice cubes

fresh mint (optional)

dash of nutmeg (optional)

1 tsp. honey (optional)

Place all ingredients except ice cubes in blender. Puree until smooth. Add ice, and puree again. Pour into a glass and sprinkle nutmeg on top and garnish the some fresh mint.

CANTALOUPE SMOOTHIE

1 Ripe banana

1/4 Ripe cantaloupe

1/2 c Nonfat or low-fat yogurt

2 tb Skim-milk powder

1 1/2 tb Orange-juice concentrate

2 ts Honey

Place unpeeled banana in the freezer overnight. Remove banana from the freezer and let it sit for 2 minutes, or until the skin begins to soften. With a paring knife, remove the skin. (Don't worry if a little fiber remains.) Cut the banana into chunks and put in a blender or food processor. Seed the cantaloupe quarter and cut the flesh from the rind. Cut the flesh into chunks and add to the blender. Add the remaining ingredients and blend until smooth. Serves 1.

CANTALOUPE BANANA SMOOTHIE

1 banana, cut in chunks and frozen
1/4 cantaloupe, cut in pieces
1/2 c nonfat yogurt
2 Tbsp. dry milk powder
1 1/2 Tbsp. orange-juice concentrate
2 tsp honey

Place all ingredients in blender and process until smooth and creamy. Serves 2.

CANTALOUPE BERRY SMOOTHIE

1/2 cantaloupe - peeled, seeded and cubed
1/2 cup plain yogurt
1 cup raspberries
3 tablespoons white sugar

In a blender, combine cantaloupe chunks, yogurt, raspberries and sugar. Blend until smooth. Pour into glasses and serve. Servers 2.

CANTALOUPE CHERRY SMOOTHIE

1/2 cantaloupe (peeled, seeded, and sliced)

1/2 cup apple or apricot juice

2-3 pitted cherries

1/4 cup raspberries or blackberries

3-4 ice cubes

Put all ingredients into blender. Blend until smoothie consistency is reached.

CARROT SMOOTHIE

2 cups carrot juice

1/2 cup apple juice

6 oz. non-fat vanilla or plain yogurt, frozen

1 banana

Put all ingredients into blender.

Blend until smoothie consistency is reached!

CHERRY VANILLA SMOOTHIE

1/4 cup Cherry Sugarfree syrup

1/4 cup Vanilla Sugarfree syrup

2 scoops VegeFuel

1 1/2 cups crushed ice

Blend until smooth.

CHOCOLATE BANANA SMOOTHIE I

1 frozen banana -- peeled

6 oz. light (reduced sugar) fat-free cherry -- frozen yogurt

2 T. Hershey's Chocolate Syrup

1/2 cup non-fat milk

Put all ingredients into blender. Blend until smoothie consistency is reached! Serves 1.

CHOCOLATE BANANA SMOOTHIE II

6 oz. SnackWell's Chocolate Cherry Non-Fat Yogurt

1/4 cup skim milk

1 banana

3 large ice cubes

Put all ingredients into blender.

Blend well, adding more ice or milk if necessary, until smoothie consistency is reached!

CHOCOLATE KITTY SMOOTHIE

1/2 bar of Heresy's milk chocolate bar
2 scoops chocolate ice cream
1/2 cup milk
ice cubes

In a blender, puree chocolate bar. Add ice cream, milk and ice cubes. Blend until smooth! Serves 2.

CHOCOLATE PEANUT BUTTER BANANA SMOOTHIE

1 banana

2 Tbs. Peanut Butter (chunky or smooth... whatever you prefer!)

1-2 squirts of Hershey's reduced calorie chocolate syrup

1 Tbs. wheat germ

6 oz. soy milk

Put all ingredients into blender.

Blend until smoothie consistency is reached!

COFFEE BANANA SMOOTHIE

2 small bananas, peeled, cut up, and frozen
1-1/2 cups skim milk
1 8-ounce container low-fat coffee yogurt
1/4 teaspoon ground cinnamon
Dash ground nutmeg
Banana slices (optional)
Fresh mint (optional)
In a blender container combine frozen bananas, milk, yogurt, cinnamon, and nutmeg. Cover and blend till smooth. To serve, pour into glasses. If desired, garnish with fresh banana slices and mint.

COLOSSAL CRANBERRY SMOOTHIE

1 1/2 cups Cran-Raspberry Juice
2 cups frozen mixed berries
1 1/2 cups nonfat vanilla frozen yogurt

Put all ingredients into blender and blend until smooth. Serves 2

CRANBERRY ORANGE SMOOTHIE

1 cup cranberry juice
1/2 cup sorbet, raspberry-flavored
1 tablespoon orange juice concentrate
1 1/2 cup orange sections
1/2 cup fresh cranberries, or cherries

Combine the cranberry juice, sorbet, and orange juice concentrate in a blender. Add the orange sections and cranberries. Blend until smooth. Serves 2

CREAMY BLUEBERRY SMOOTHIE

6 oz. light (reduced sugar) fat-free blueberry yogurt, frozen

(This is one container of Yoplait)

1 cup blueberries, fresh

1 cup non-fat milk

Put all ingredients into blender. Blend until smoothie consistency is reached! 1/2 cup frozen blueberries may be added to make it thicker.

FAST TRACK BREAKFAST SMOOTHIE

16 oz Low Fat Blueberry Or Strawberry Yogurt
1 1/4 C Skim Milk
3/4 C Fresh Or Frozen Blueberries Or Strawberries
3 Tbsp Dry Milk Powder
2 Tsp Honey
In a blender, blend until smooth. Good health: lower cholesterol, stronger immunity, makes 4. Can be frozen, leave in frig. to thaw overnight, stir well before drinking.

FAT FREE CANTALOUPE SMOOTHIE

1/2 ripe cantaloupe, peeled, seeded, and cut into chunks
1 cup (250 ml) skim milk
1 cup (250 ml) unflavored or vanilla fat-free yogurt
1 cup (250 ml) crushed ice
2 Tbs (30 ml) sugar, or to taste
Combine all ingredients in an electric blender and process until smooth. Serves 2.

FRESH FRUIT SMOOTHIE

1 Cup Watermelon; Cut Up

1 Cup Cantaloupe Or Honeydew;

1 Cup Pineapple; Cut Up

1 Cup Mango; Cut Up

1 Cup Strawberries; Halved

1/4 Cup Sugar

1 Cup Orange Juice

Crushed Ice

Mix all ingredients except ice. Fill blender container 1/2 full of mixture. Add crushed ice to fill to the top. Cover and blend on high speed until of a uniform consistency. Repeat with remaining mixture. Serve immediately; garnish with fruit, if desired. Serves 6.

FROSTIE FRUIT SMOOTHIE

3/4 cup chilled pineapple juice
1 cup fresh strawberries
1 ripe banana
ice cubes

Place all ingredients in blender. Process until smooth.

FROZEN BANANA SMOOTHIE

2 frozen bananas

Vanilla extract

Sliced seasonal fruit

Cut frozen banana into 4 pieces and cut away peel and discard. In blender, blend banana until thick and smooth. Add a dash of vanilla extract and blend again. Scoop out and serve with fresh sliced seasonal fruit.

FROZEN FRUIT SMOOTHIE

For the fruit:

choose a mix from below

Frozen strawberries

Frozen banana slices

Frozen raspberries

Frozen blueberries

Frozen peach slices

Sugar to taste

For the flavoring =(choose one):

Vanilla extract = 1/2 teaspoon per batch

Chocolate syrup = 2 tablespoons per batch

For the liquid = (choose one):

Milk

Orange juice

Flavored yogurt = peach/vanilla/ lemon etc

In a blender combine the fruit with the sugar, the chosen flavoring and enough of the chosen liquid to barely cover the fruit. Blend until smooth. Taste to adjust seasoning. Garnish with a strawberry and a sprig of mint.

FRUIT CREAM SMOOTHIE

1/2 c nonfat vanilla yogurt

1/4 c skim milk

1 banana -- frozen

1/2 c raspberries, frozen

1/2 c strawberries, frozen

1 tbsp maple syrup

Combine all in blender or food processor until smooth.

FRUIT 'N' HONEY SMOOTHIE

1 Scoop Vanilla frozen yogurt

8 ounces apple juice frozen

fresh fruit

a squeeze of honey

ice

Blend in blender until smooth Serves 1.

FRUIT SALAD SMOOTHIE

1 md Ripe peach

3/4 c Fresh OR frozen strawberries

1/2 Banana -- peeled

2 c Skimmed evaporated milk -chilled

4 ts Frozen orange juice concentrate

1 t Vanilla

4-6 ice cubes

Cinnamon -- optional

Combine everything in blender except ice and cinnamon. With blender running, add ice cubes one at a time. Divide Smoothie into 4 chilled glasses and sprinkle with cinnamon. Serves 4.

FRUIT SMOOTHIE I

1 banana, peeled, cut in half, and frozen
4 or 5 frozen strawberries, stem removed
1 six ounce container strawberry or strawberry/banana yogurt
Let frozen banana and strawberries thaw for 5 to 10 minutes on counter top. Add all ingredients to blender. Pulse the blender button until you can tell the ingredients have all been chopped smooth. Makes approximately 2, eight-oz. servings.

FRUIT SMOOTHIE II

8 oz Fruit cocktail, can, chilled

1 c Milk

1/4 c Nonfat dry milk powder

1/2 ts Vanilla

1/2 c Ice cubes

2 x Cinnamon, ground (dashes)

In a blender container combine undrained fruit cocktail and remaining ingredients. Cover; blend till combined. Add ice cubes; cover and blend till smooth. Sprinkle with additional cinnamon (for garnish), if desired. Serve immediately. Serves 4.

FRUIT SPICE SMOOTHIE

1 frozen banana (best if cut into 1-inch chunks, then frozen)

1/2 - 1 cup hulled strawberries (don't need to cut them up)

1/4 - 1/2 cup soy milk, orange juice, or water cinnamon to taste

Add all of the ingredients in a blender. I start with 1/4 cup of liquid and add more depending on how thick I want the smoothie. Blend in spurts until smooth. Variations: * Use peaches, blueberries, apple slices, or more bananas in place of strawberries (or combine them!) May need to vary the liquid depending on the juiciness of the fruit. * Use fresh bananas and 1-2 ice cubes * In addition to the cinnamon, add one or more of: nutmeg, cloves, ginger, vanilla

FRUITY BANANA SMOOTHIE

6-8 oz plain yogurt

½ banana

1 cup of frozen fruit (usually strawberries, raspberries, and/or blueberries)

4-5 oz plain soy milk

a dash of vanilla

1 teaspoon of honey

Blend it all up.

FUZZY BANANA NAVEL

(serves 4)

2 medium bananas quartered
1 pint orange sorbet or 2 cups orange sherbet, slightly softened
1 cup Mandarin Tangerine juice

Combine bananas, sorbet and juice in blender container. Blend until thick and smooth. Garnish with orange slices and curls. Serve immediately.

GALA APPLE SMOOTHIE

1 Gala apple, peeled, cored and chopped
1 frozen banana, peeled and chopped
1/2 cup orange juice
1/4 cup nonfat milk

In a blender combine frozen banana, orange juice, apple and milk. Blend until smooth. pour into glasses and serve. Makes 2 servings

GETTIN' MY GROOVE BACK SMOOTHIE

1 cup of natural orange juice

1 cup of sliced strawberries

2 mangos peeled and with seeds removed

2 tablespoons of Grade B Maple syrup

1/3 teaspoon of Cinnamon

¼ Tablespoon of vanilla extract

1 cup of crushed ice

Place all ingredients in blender, mix and drink

GINGER TROPICAL SMOOTHIE

1/2 cup orange juice
1/4 cup pineapple juice
1/2 banana
1/4 to 1/2 tsp grated fresh ginger root
1/2 cup crushed ice, or 2 small ice cubes

Add all ingredients to blender and process until smooth.

Serves 1

GRAPE EXPLOSION SMOOTHIE

2 cups red seedless grapes
1 cup green seedless grapes
1/2 cup purple grape juice
2 teaspoons lime juice
1 teaspoon peeled and minced fresh gingerroot
3 ice cubes

Combine all ingredients in blender and whip until smooth.

Serves 2

HAWAIIAN HOLIDAY SMOOTHIE

1 cup passion fruit nectar
1 cup guava nectar
1 cup orange sherbet
4 Tbs. coconut milk
1/2 frozen banana in chunks
1/2 cup frozen strawberries
1/2 cup frozen mango slices
1 cup strawberry yogurt Pour all liquid ingredients into the blender. Add all frozen ingredients. Blend at MIX setting for 30 seconds then blend at SMOOTH setting until smooth. While the machine is running, move the stir stick around counter-clockwise to aid mixing. Serve immediately. Each recipe serves 3-5.

HAWAIIAN SMOOTHIE

1 cup cubed peeled pineapple
1 cup cubed peeled papaya
1/2 cup pineapple juice or papaya nectar
1 ripe banana (about 6 oz.), peeled and cut into chunks
1/2 cup nonfat vanilla yogurt
1/8 to 1/4 teaspoon coconut extract

Combine all ingredients in blender and blend until smooth.

Serves 2

HAWAIIAN SILK SMOOTHIE

1 cup soy milk

1/2 cup pineapple juice

1 frozen banana

1 Tbs. maple syrup

2 Tbs. nonfat dry milk

Ice cubes

1 Tbs. coconut milk

Put all ingredients into blender.

Blend until smoothie consistency is reached!

HEALING SMOOTHIE

1 firm kiwi fruit -- peeled

1/4 cantaloupe -- with skin

1 ripe banana

Push kiwi fruit and cantaloupe through the hopper. Place juice and banana in a blender or food processor and blend until smooth. Pour into a tall glass, drink immediately and enjoy!! This is a great drink for anyone, especially those with ulcers. This drink has soothing qualities which protect and heal the stomach lining. Serves 1.

HEALTHY SMOOTHIE

2 C. yogurt (Plain)
1 C. orange juice
1 C. grapes (essential for sweetness)
1 apple
1 or 2 sm. bananas
12 walnuts
1 bale shredded wheat or ½ C. Grape Nuts
To these basic ingredients add/subtract: 2 C. sugar-free frozen fruit, 1 orange, 1 peach, 8 oz. dried apricots (can be soaked in the orange juice), 1 kiwi, cantaloupe/honeydew melon (in season). Place all in a blender and blend at high speed.

HI FIBER BERRY SMOOTHIE

1 cup blackberries
1 cup stemmed and halved strawberries
1 cup blueberries
1 cup low-fat vanilla soymilk
1/8 teaspoon ground cinnamon
3 ice cubes

Combine all ingredients in blender and whip until smooth. If berries are not fully ripe, add a little honey or sugar substitute for sweetness.

serves 2

HIGH PROTEIN SMOOTHIE

1 cup Vanilla honey ice milk

1 cup milk

1 Banana -- peeled and cut in chunks

3 Pecans -- broken

2 tablespoons wheat germ

2 tablespoons Protein powder

Combine ice milk, raw milk, banana, pecans, wheat germ, and protein powder in b lender container. Blend until smooth but still thick. Pour into chilled glass. Serves 1.

ISLAND FRUIT SMOOTHIE

1 small banana, peeled and cut into chunks
2 tablespoons coconut milk
2 tablespoons lime juice
1/4 cup orange juice
1/4 cup pineapple juice
1/2 teaspoon ginger, grated
3 ice cubes

In a blender, blend all ingredients until smooth. Yield: 1 smoothie

JADE ZINGER SMOOTHIE

1 cucumber, peeled, seeded and chopped

3 tablespoons mint leaves & mint spigs -- finely chopped

1 1/2 cups apple juice or still cider

1 cup lemon sorbet

1 cup ice cubes

Place the cucumber, mint, apple juice or cider, sorbet and ice in a blender, and blend until smooth. Garnish with mint, and serve. Yield: 2 16-ounce servings.

KIWI COOLER SMOOTHIE

1 1/2 cups diced fresh kiwi
1 1/2 cups lime sherbet
1 cup diced ripe banana
1 cup honeydew melon
Place all ingredients in a blender or food processor. Process until smooth. Serves 3

KIWI LIME SMOOTHIE

2 kiwi fruit

1 banana

1 teaspoon lime juice

1/2 teaspoon grated lime zest

2 ice cubes

1 cup skim milk

1/4 cup part skim millk

ricotta cheese

Peel kiwifruits and banana; cut into large chunks. Place fruit, lime juice, lime zest and ice cubes in food processor or blender; process until blended. Add milk and ricotta; process for another 5-10 seconds, scraping down sides of container with rubber spatula. Pour shake into 2 tall glasses and serve. Serve 2.

KIWI STRAWBERRY SMOOTHIE

3 peeled kiwi

1 cup frozen banana slices

3/4 cup pineapple juice

1/2 cup frozen strawberries

Put all ingredients into blender. Blend until smoothie consistency is reached!

LEMON APPLE HONEY SMOOTHIE

1/4 cup lemon juice
1/2 cup apple cider
1 apple (about 8 oz.), peeled, cored, and chopped
1 peeled banana
2 to 3 tablespoons honey
1 cup nonfat or vanilla frozen yogurt

Combine in blender till smooth.

Serves 2

LEMON LOUIE SMOOTHIE

2 cups lemonade
1 cup lemon yogurt
1 1/2 cups frozen pineapple chunks
1 cup pineapple sherbet Pour all liquid ingredients into the blender. Add all frozen ingredients. Blend at MIX setting for 30 seconds then blend at SMOOTH setting until smooth. While the machine is running, move the stir stick around counter-clockwise to aid mixing. Serve immediately. Each recipe serves 3-5.

LEMON MELON SMOOTHIE

1 1/2 cups diced honeydew melon
1/2 cup nonfat lemon yogurt
1 cup frozen green grapes
1 tablespoon chopped fresh mint
Fresh lemon juice to taste (optional)

Combine the honeydew melon and lemon yogurt in a blender. Add the grapes and mint. Blend until smooth. Taste and add lemon juice if you like.

Serves 2

LEMON PEACH SMOOTHIE

1 Dannon Lit N Fit Lemon Chiffon Yogurt
1 Fresh Peach or 1 small can of lite canned peaches
2 - 4 Ice Cubes

Place all in blender and blend till Smooth. Add a dash of nutmeg on top and enjoy!

Serves 1

LEMON STRAWBERRY YOGURT SMOOTHIE

1 cup nonfat vanilla yogurt
1/2 cup orange juice
1 1/2 cup strawberries
1/2 cup crushed ice
1 T. lemon juice
1/2 tsp. lemon zest

Combine all in blender until smooth.

Serves 1 (large)

LIMEY MELON SMOOTHIE

1 1/2 cups watermelon – chopped
1 1/2 cups honeydew melon – chopped
2 limes -- juice only
1 cup vanilla lowfat yogurt
1 cup ice cubes
Place all ingredients in a blender and blend until smooth. Pour into glasses.
Yield: 4 serving

LOTS O FRUIT SMOOTHIE

All begin with a base of:
½ c. plain, vanilla, or strawberry yogurt
¼-1/2 c. milk
then perhaps some fruit juice, usually orange or Dole specialty juices, ¼-1/2c.
Followed by fruit in many varying combinations, always including either banana or melon.
1 banana
handful frozen or fresh strawberries or
blueberries
one 4-5" wide slice out of a cantaloupe or
honeydew melon
1 kiwi
Then I'd blend it till I was pleased with the result. I found that melon added a lot of sweetness and made a nice background taste. I don't always use juice when I use the melon. We especially liked melon and blueberries, bananas and strawberries.

MACHO POWER SMOOTHIE

1 cup nonfat soy milk (such as Healthy Valley Soy Moo)

1/2 cup orange juice

1 banana

1/2 cup cantaloupe

1 T. peanut butter

1/2 cup strawberries, fresh or frozen (without sugar)

Put all ingredients into blender.

Blend well until smoothie consistency is reached!

MAIN SQUEEZE SMOOTHIE

1 1/2 cups ripe strawberries, hulled and sliced
1 cup raspberries
1 banana, peeled and sliced
1 cup orange juice (preferably freshly squeezed)

Place all ingredients in blender and process until smooth.

Serves 2

MALTED DATE SMOOTHIE

1/2 cup pitted dates

1/2 cup nonfat milk
3 tablespoons malt powder
1 1/2 cups nonfat vanilla frozen yogurt

Combine all ingredients in blender and blend until smooth.

Serves 2

MANGO SMOOTHIE I

1/2 cup orange juice
1/2 cup peeled, pitted and sliced fresh mango
honey to taste
1/2 cup ice
Place the juice, fruit and honey in a blender. Blend on high speed for 30 seconds. Add the ice and blend until smooth.

MANGO SMOOTHIE II

1 ripe mango, peeled, pitted, chopped -- (approx. 1-1/4 cups)

3/4 cup milk, skim -- chilled

1/4 cup nonfat vanilla yogurt

3/4 teaspoon vanilla extract

3 ice cubes

pinch of salt

fresh mint sprigs

Combine all ingredients except mint in blender. Blend until smooth and creamy. Garnish with mint. Serves 1.

MANGO GINGER SMOOTHIE

2 ripe mangoes, peeled and chopped
2 pieces crystallized ginger, about 1 ounce
1 cup nonfat buttermilk
One 8-ounce container nonfat vanilla yogurt
Handful of chipped ice

In a blender, purée the fruit and ginger, scraping down the sides as necessary. Add the buttermilk, yogurt and ice and purée until smooth and frothy.

Serves 2

MANGO MANIA SMOOTHIE

2 cups nonfat vanilla yogurt
1 cup mango nectar
2 mangos, peeled and chopped
1/4 tsp. cardomom

Add all ingredients to blender and process until smooth. Add 1 cup of ice cubes and blend till crushed and smooth.

Serves 2

MANGO PEACH SMOOTHIE

1 cup peeled mango chunks
1 large peach (about 8 oz.), peeled, pitted, and cut into chunks
1 cup peach nectar
2 tablespoons lime juice

Combine all ingredients in blender and blend until smooth.

Makes two small drinks.

MANGO TANGO SMOOTHIE

1 cup pineapple juice
1 cup orange juice
1/2 frozen banana (chunks)
1 cup pineapple sherbet
1 1/2 cups frozen mango slices Pour all liquid ingredients into the blender. Add all frozen ingredients. Blend at MIX setting for 30 seconds then blend at SMOOTH setting until smooth. While the machine is running, move the stir stick around counter-clockwise to aid mixing. Serve immediately. Each recipe serves 3-5.

MEGA SMOOTHIE

1 mango -- peeled, seeded and chopped

2 bananas -- peeled and chopped

8 large strawberries

2 medium carrots -- chopped

2 cups ice cubes

1 tablespoon honey

1 cup yogurt -- optional

In a blender combine half of each ingredient, including: mango, bananas, strawberries, carrots, ice cubes, honey and yogurt and blend until smooth. Pour into a glass and serve immediately. Repeat process for remaining ingredients. Yield: 2 servings

MELON MADNESS SMOOTHIE

1 1/2 cups seeded and chopped watermelon
1 1/2 cups seeded and chopped honeydew melon
Juice of 2 limes
1 cup vanilla nonfat yogurt
1 cup ice cubes

Place all ingredients in a blender and blend until smooth. Pour into glasses.

Makes 4 servings

MELON MINT SMOOTHIE

2 cups diced cantaloupe
1 cup diced honeydew melon
1 cup diced seedless watermelon
1/2 cup passion fruit or mango juice
1 tablespoon lime juice
2 teaspoons honey
10 fresh mint leaves
3 ice cubes

Combine all ingredients in blender and whip until smooth.

Serves 2

MELON SMOOTHIE

1 1/2 cups seeded and chopped watermelon
1 1/2 cups seeded and chopped honeydew melon
Juice of 2 limes
1 cup vanilla lowfat yogurt
1 cup ice cubes
Place all ingredients in a blender and blend until smooth. Pour into glasses. Yield: 4 servings

MORNING SUNRISE SMOOTHIE

(serves 1)

1 Banana, peeled and sliced
1/2 cup of strawberries
1/2 cup of orange juice
A handful of ice cubes

Place all ingredients in blender and blend until smooth.

MUCHO MELON SMOOTHIE

1 cup of peach fat-free yogurt, frozen

1 cup skim milk

1/2 cup cantaloupe

1/2 cup honey dew melon

4 ice cubes

1/2 cup strawberries (or substitute with watermelon)

Put yogurt, milk, and strawberries into blender. Blend on high for about 30-45 seconds. Then add in cantaloupe, melon, and ice. Blend once again on high for 1 minute.

NECTARINE SMOOTHIE

1/4 cup orange juice
1/2 cup plain, low-fat yogurt
1/2 cup peeled, pitted and sliced nectarines
honey to taste
Place all the ingredients in a blender. Blend on high speed until smooth.

NECTARINE BERRY SMOOTHIE

1 nectarine, pitted
3/4 cup strawberries, hulled
3/4 cup blueberries, rinsed and drained
1/3 cup nonfat dry milk powder
1 cup crushed ice

In a blender combine nectarine, strawberries, blueberries, milk powder and crushed ice. Blend until smooth. pour into glasses and serve.

serves 2

NON-FAT LOW CALORIE STRAWBERRY BANANA SMOOTHIE

Maui Wowi
Recipe for a refreshing day-If you can't get a Maui Wowi, here is the next best thing.
1 Cup Fresh Strawberries
1 Banana
1 cup Non-fat yogurt
1 packet sugar or sugar substitute
2 cups ice
Blend until creamy

O LAWD IN A GLASS SMOOTHIE

½ cup of sliced strawberries

2 apples peeled, cut and with seeds removed

½ cup of blueberries

½ cup of peaches

¾ cup of natural apple juice

¾ cup of natural orange juice

Place all ingredients in blender, mix and drink

Make sure your juices are not from concentrate

ORANGE BANANA CREAM SMOOTHIE

1/4 cup orange juice
1/4 cup pineapple juice
1 tbsp coconut milk
1/2 banana
1/4 tsp grated fresh ginger root
1/2 cup crushed ice or 2 small ice cubes

Add all ingredients to blender and process until smooth. Serves 1.

ORANGE FRUITY SMOOTHIE

1 medium banana, peeled and cut into 1-inch pieces
1 ripe peach, peeled, halved, pitted, and diced
1 cup raspberries
1 1/2 cups freshly squeezed orange juice
3 ice cubes

Combine all ingredients in blender and whip until smooth. Serves 2

ORANGE PINEAPPLE COCONUT SMOOTHIE

1/4 cup orange juice
1/4 cup pineapple juice
1 tbsp coconut milk
1/2 banana
1/4 tsp grated fresh ginger root
1/2 cup crushed ice or 2 small ice cubes

Add all ingredients to blender and process until smooth. Serves 1.

ORANGE PINEAPPLE GINGER SMOOTHIE

1/2 c Orange juice

1/4 c Pineapple juice

1/2 ea Banana

1/4 ts Ginger root -- fresh,peeled, -grated, up to 1/2 tsp

1/2 c -Crushed ice -- or 2 small ice -cubes

Blend all until smooth.

ORANGE SMOOTHIE I

2 oranges, peeled & sectioned
1 frozen banana, chunked
¼ c. orange juice
2 T. yogurt
1 tsp. vanilla Blend in blender until smooth. Serves 2.

ORANGE SMOOTHIE II

6 oz Orange juice concentrate -- frozen

1 c Milk

1 c Water

1/4 c Sugar

1/2 ts Vanilla

10 Ice cubes

Place all ingredients in a blender. Cover and blend until smooth. Serve immediately. Serves 6.

ORANGE FRUITY SMOOTHIE

1 medium banana, peeled and cut into 1-inch pieces
1 ripe peach, peeled, halved, pitted, and diced
1 cup raspberries
1 1/2 cups freshly squeezed orange juice

3 ice cubes

Combine all ingredients in blender and whip until smooth.

Serves 2

PAPAYA CREAMSICLE SMOOTHIE

2 ea Papayas; ripe

1/2 c Orange juice

1/2 c Vanilla frozen yogurt

Peel, seed and coarsely chop papayas. Combine all ingredients in a blender or food processor and blend until smooth.

PAPAYA SMOOTHIE

1/2 cup orange juice
3/4 cup peeled, seeded and chopped ripe papaya
honey to taste
1/2 cup ice
Place the juice, fruit and honey in a blender. Blend on high speed for 30 seconds. Add the ice and blend until smooth.

PAPAYA BERRY SMOOTHIE

1 frozen banana (freezing it makes the drink super cold without diluting it with ice)

1/2 fresh papaya

10-12 raspberries (fresh or frozen)

1/2 c water or fruit juice

1 tbsp toasted wheat germ (optional)

Puree in blender 30-45 seconds. makes about sixteen delicious, filling, vegan, nutritious ounces.

PAPAYA NECTARINE SMOOTHIE

1 cup Crystal Light or any other sugar-free lemonade

6 oz. fat free peach yogurt, frozen

(This is one container of Yoplait)

1 nectarine, pitted and unpeeled

1 cup papaya, seeded and peeled

Put all ingredients into blender. Blend well until smoothie consistency is reached!

PAPAYA RASPBERRY SMOOTHIE

1 frozen banana, peeled

1/2 fresh papaya

10-12 raspberries (fresh or frozen)

1/2 cup water or fruit juice

Put all ingredients into blender. Blend until smoothie consistency is reached!

PEACH BERRY SMOOTHIE

1 cup nonfat peach yogurt
3/4 cup peach nectar
1/2 cup raspberries
1 1/2 cup ripe medium peaches, diced

Combine the yogurt and nectar in a blender. Add the raspberries and peaches. Blend until smooth.

Serves 2

PEACH CINNAMON SMOOTHIE

2 ripe peaches
2 cups nonfat plain yogurt
3 tablespoons firmly packed brown sugar
1/4 teaspoon ground cinnamon
1 cup ice cubes

In a 2- to 3-quart pan over high heat, bring about 1 quart water to a boil. Immerse peaches in boiling water for 15 seconds; drain. When peaches are cool enough to touch, in 1 to 2 minutes, peel, pit, and cut into chunks. In a blender, combine peaches, yogurt, brown sugar, and cinnamon; whirl on high speed until smooth, about 1 minute. Add ice and whirl until smooth, about 2 minutes longer. Pour into tall glasses (at least 16-oz. size).

Serves 2

PEACH MELBA SMOOTHIE

1 cup peeled, sliced peaches

1/4 cup fresh or frozen raspberries
1 cup chilled peach juice
1/2 vanilla yogurt
3 ice cubes

Pour all items in a blender and blend until smooth. Pour into 2 glasses and garnish with fruit. Serves 2.

PEACH REFRESHER

2 cups peach nectar or apple juice
1 cup vanilla frozen yogurt
1/2 banana
1 cup peach yogurt
1 1/2 cups frozen peach slices Pour all liquid ingredients into the blender. Add all frozen ingredients. Blend at MIX setting for 30 seconds then blend at SMOOTH setting until smooth. While the machine is running, move the stir stick around counter-clockwise to aid mixing. Serve immediately. Each recipe serves 3-5.

PEACHES & CRANBERRY SMOOTHIE

1 can peaches

1 cup cranberry juice

½ cup plain yogurt

1 cup crushed ice

Strain off juice from large can of peaches and throw juice away. Blend until smooth. Serves 4.

PEACHY APPLE SMOOTHIE

1 fresh peach

1/3 cup non-fat milk

1/4 cup of frozen apple juice concentrate

Peal 1 fresh peach. Cut it into thin slices. Put into a plastic bag with a zipper bag, laying flat. Put the plastic bag into the freezer for 1-2 hours. Take out 1/4 of the peaches and break them into pieces. Mix in a blender with 1/3 cup of milk and 1/4 cup of frozen apple juice concentrate. Cover and blend until smooth. pour into a glass, and add more peach slices for peachy ice cubes!

PEACHY BLUE SMOOTHIE

1 peach, frozen

10 blueberries, frozen

1 cup light (reduced sugar) fat-free vanilla yogurt, frozen

1/2 cup 1% milk

1/2 T. crushed pecan

1/2 tsp salt

1/4 tsp vanilla extract

Put all ingredients into blender. Blend until smoothie consistency is reached!

PEACHY COOLER SMOOTHIE

1 c Chilled peach nectar
½ c Milk
1 Container (6 ounces) peach yogurt
Ground nutmeg
Place nectar, milk and yogurt in blender. Cover and blend on high speed about 30 seconds or until smooth. Sprinkle with nutmeg. 2 servings (about 1-1/4 cups each); 180 calories per serving.

PEACHY POWER SMOOTHIE

1 cup Low-fat vanilla yogurt

1 cup Sliced peaches

1/4 cup Wheat germ

1/4 cup Orange juice

1 cup Ice cubes

In blender or food processor, combine yogurt, peaches, banana, wheat germ,= 1/4 cup orange juice and ice cubes. Cover and blend about 1 minute, or until smooth. Serve immediately, poured into tall glasses and garnished with peach slices and sprinkled with 2 tablespoons wheat germ.

PEACHY PUNCH SMOOTHIE

10 oz of apple cider

3-5 slices of peach

4 large strawberries

1 banana

1/8 tsp of cinnamon

Put all ingredients into blender. Blend well until smoothie consistency is reached!

PEANUT BUTTER BANANA SMOOTHIE

1 banana, frozen, cut in chunks
2 Tbsp. reduced fat creamy peanut butter
1 cup skim milk
1/2 cup frozen vanilla yogurt or fat free ice cream

Mix in blender till smooth. Serves 2.

PEANUT BUTTER POWER SMOOTHIE

1/2 cup soy milk

1/2 cup silken tofu

1/3 cup creamy peanut butter

2 bananas -- frozen

2 tablespoons chocolate syrup

Combine soy milk, tofu, and peanut butter in blender. Add bananas, chocolate syrup, and any ice cubes if desired. Blend until smooth. Serves 2.

PEANUT BUTTER SUNDAE SMOOTHIE

1/4 cup smooth peanut butter

2 Tablespoons honey

1/3 cup milk

3 cups vanilla ice milk

1/4 teaspoon wheat germ

Stir peanut butter, honey and milk together. Cook over low heat, stirring constantly. Remove from heat when peanut butter has melted; stir in ice milk and wheat germ; serve chilled. Serves 4.

PEAR SMOOTHIE

1 1/2 c. diced pears
1/2 c. peach yogurt
1/2 c. pear nectar

1 tsp. lemon juice
1/4 tsp. grated fresh ginger
3-5 ice cubes

PINA COLADA SMOOTHIE I

5 Tbs. Coconut milk
2 1/2 cups pineapple juice
1/2 cup vanilla ice cream
1/2 frozen banana (chunks)
1 1/2 cups frozen pineapple chunks Pour all liquid ingredients into the blender. Add all frozen ingredients. Blend at MIX setting for 30 seconds then blend at SMOOTH setting until smooth. While the machine is running, move the stir stick around counter-clockwise to aid mixing. Serve immediately. Each recipe serves 3-5.

PINA COLADA SMOOTHIE II

1 6oz container nonfat coconut yogurt (frozen)

1/2 banana (frozen)

1/2 of a 20 oz can crushed pineapple

1 c. nonfat milk

Put all ingredients into blender. Blend well until smoothie consistency is reached!

PINA COLADA SLUSH SMOOTHIE

2 cups cubed fresh pineapple
1-1/2 cups pineapple juice, chilled
1/4 cup cream of coconut (such as Coco Lopez)
1 cup ice cubes
1 cup vanilla fat-free frozen yogurt
Place pineapple into freezer; freeze until firm (about 1 hour). Remove from freezer; let stand 10 minutes. Combine juice and cream in a blender. With blender on, add pineapple and ice cubes, 1 at a time; process until smooth. Add yogurt; process until smooth. Serve immediately.

PINEAPPLE SMOOTHIE

20 oz Unsweetened pineapple chunks

1 c Buttermilk

2 ts Vanilla extract

2 ts Liquid sweetener

Mint Leaves--Optional

Drain pineapple, reserving 1/2 cup juice. Freeze pineapple chunks. Place juice, buttermilk, vanilla, sweetener and frozen pineapple into a blender container. Blend until smooth. Pour into glasses and garnish with mint if desired.

PINEAPPLE BERRY SMOOTHIE

1 cup orange juice

1/4 cup pineapple juice

2 pineapple rings (Dole pineapple slices)

6 fresh strawberries

12-15 frozen raspberries

8-10 frozen boysenberries

12-15 frozen blueberries

3 oz. non-fat yogurt, any flavor (about half a container of Yoplait)

Ice (however much you prefer for consistency)

Put all ingredients into blender. Blend well until smoothie consistency is reached!

PINEAPPLE CANTALOUPE SMOOTHIE

1 1/2 cups diced pineapple
1 1/2 cups diced cantaloupe
1/2 cup freshly squeezed orange juice
1/2 cup carrot juice
Pinch nutmeg
3 ice cubes

Combine all ingredients in blender and whip until smooth. Serves 2.

PINEAPPLE COCONUT SMOOTHIE

1/2 cup buttermilk
1 cup pineapple chunks, canned in juice, drained
1 tsp. coconut flakes
1/2 tsp. coconut extract

Add all ingredients to blender and process until smooth. Serves 1.

PINEAPPLE DELIGHT SMOOTHIE

2 cups nonfat milk
2 bananas, frozen and chunked
6 slices canned pineapple

1 tablespoon honey

In a blender combine milk, frozen bananas, pineapple and honey. Blend until smooth. Makes 4 cups, or 2 large servings.

PINEAPPLE ORANGE BANANA SMOOTHIE

1 banana

6 oz. light (reduced sugar) fat-free peach yogurt, frozen

(This is one container of Yoplait)

6 oz. (1 can) Dole Pine-Orange-Banana juice

Put all ingredients into blender. Blend until smoothie consistency is reached! If drink is too thick, add orange juice.

PINEAPPLE PAPAYA SMOOTHIE

1/2 cup orange juice
1/4 cup peeled, cored and cubed pineapple
1/4 cup peeled, seeded and chopped ripe papaya
honey to taste
1/2 cup ice
Place the juice, fruit and honey in a blender. Blend on high speed for 30 seconds. Add the ice and blend until smooth.

PISTACHIO BANANA SMOOTHIE

1 container plain nonfat yogurt

2-3 oz pistachio instant pudding mix

1 ripe banana

1/4 c skim milk

handful or more of crushed ice

Put all ingredients into blender. Blend until smoothie consistency is reached!

POWER BERRY SMOOTHIE

1 cup cranberry juice
1 cup fresh or frozen strawberries
1 8 ounce container of vanilla yogurt
2/3 cup uncooked oats
1 cup ice cubes
sugar to taste

Place all ingredients except ice in blender. Cover and blend on high for 2 minutes or until smooth. Gradually add ice cubes; blend on high until smooth.

Serve immediately.

POWER FRUIT SMOOTHIE

1 frozen banana (best if cut into 1-inch -- chunks then f rozen)

1/2 cup hulled strawberries (don't need to cut them up)

1/4 cup soy milk, orange juice or water

cinnamon to taste

Add all of the ingredients in a blender. I start with 1/4 cup of liquid and add more depending on how thick I want the smoothie. Blend in spurts until smooth. Variations: * Use peaches, blueberries, apple slices, or more bananas in place of strawberries (or combine them!) May need to vary the liquid depending on the juciness of the fruit. * Use fresh bananas and 1-2 ice cubes * In addition to the cinnamon, add one or more of: nutmeg, cloves, ginger, vanilla kwvegan vegan Serves 1.

POWER SMOOTHIE

In a blender, combine 1/2 banana, 1/2 cup yogurt (I like vanilla flavored), 1/2 cup fruit juice (i.e. orange, cranberry, etc.). For added nutrition I use 1 Tbls. soy protein powder, 1 Tbls. molasses, and 1 tsp. wheat germ. Blend until smooth. Then add frozen fruit, i.e. strawberries, raspberries, etc., one at a time, until smoothie is consistency you desire.
The basic recipe is: ice, fruit, yoghurt, juice and/or milk. (I usually stick to juice, but sometimes add just a splash of milk to smooth it out.)

PUMPKIN SMOOTHIE

1 3/4 cups pumpkin, canned -- chilled
12 ounces evaporated skim milk -- chilled
1 1/2 cups orange juice
1/2 cup banana -- sliced
1/3 cup brown sugar, packed

Place all ingredients in blender and blend well. If desired, serve over ice and sprinkle with cinnamon. Serves 6.

RAINFOREST FUSION SMOOTHIE

1 cup frozen pineapple pieces
1/2 banana
1/2 cup orange juice
2 Tbsp. coconut milk
1/2 tsp. lime juice
1/2 cup nonfat frozen vanilla yogurt
1/2 cup ice

Combine ingredients in blender; mix until smooth and frothy. Serves 1.

RASPBERRY CAPPUCCINO SMOOTHIE

3/4 cup chocolate milk, low-fat
1/3 cup fresh-brewed espresso
2 tablespoon chocolate syrup
1 1/2 cup nonfat coffee flavor frozen yogurt
1 cup raspberries
1/2 cup skim milk
1/4 teaspoon cocoa powder

Combine the chocolate milk, espresso, and chocolate syrup in a blender. Add the frozen yogurt and raspberries. Blend until smooth. Pour into glasses. Rinse out the blender container. Pour the milk into the blender and blend on high speed until frothy, about 15 seconds. Divide between the smoothies and sprinkle them with chocolate powder. Serves 2.

RASPBERRY CREAM SMOOTHIE

1 cup orange juice
1 cup raspberry yogurt
1 cup vanilla frozen yogurt
1/2 frozen banana (chunks)
1 1/2 cup frozen raspberries Pour all liquid ingredients into the blender. Add all frozen ingredients. Blend at MIX setting for 30 seconds then blend at SMOOTH setting until smooth. While the machine is running, move the stir stick around counter-clockwise to aid mixing. Serve immediately. Each recipe serves 3-5.

RASPBERRY PEACH BREAKFAST SMOOTHIE

10 oz Frozen Raspberries (Frozen raspberries should be thawed and in light syrup)

1 c Canned Peach Nectar

1/2 c Buttermilk

1 tb Honey

Place all ingredients in a blender bowl and process until smooth. Pour into glasses and serve. Serves 4.

RASPBERRY PEACH SMOOTHIE

10 oz frozen raspberries (in light syrup, thawed)
1 cup peach nectar
1/2 cup buttermilk
1 Tbsp. honey

Place all ingredients in a blender and process until smooth. Serves 2.

RASPBERRY SMOOTHIE (LOW FAT)

1 pkt Weight Watchers Vanilla Smoothie
1 cup cold skim milk
1/2 cup fresh or frozen raspberries
5 ice cubes

Crush ice cubes in blender. Add smoothie mix and milk and blend. Add raspberries and frappe. If needed, add a packet or two of sugar substitute. Serves 1.

RASPBERRY SMOOTHIE I

1/4 cup orange juice
1/2 cup plain, low-fat yogurt
1/2 cup washed, stemmed raspberries
honey to taste
Place all the ingredients in a blender. Blend on high speed until smooth.

RASPBERRY SMOOTHIE II

1 cup milk
½ cup natural yogurt
1 cup raspberries
sugar or honey to taste.
Blend all ingredients on high until smooth. Pour into glasses.

RASPBERRY SUNRISE SMOOTHIE

2 1/2 cups orange juice
1 1/2 cups frozen raspberries
1 cup raspberry sherbet Pour all liquid ingredients into the blender. Add all frozen ingredients. Blend at MIX setting for 30 seconds then blend at SMOOTH setting until smooth. While the machine is running, move the stir stick around counter-clockwise to aid mixing. Serve immediately. Each recipe serves 3-5.

QUICK START BREAKFAST DRINK

2 C. Pineapple Juice
2 ripe med. bananas, peeled & sliced
2 (8 oz.) cartons vanilla yogurt
1 C. fresh or frozen strawberries
¼ C. wheat germ (opt.)
1 T. vanilla extract
Combine all ingredients in blender. Whir until smooth. (For small blender, do ½ at a time.) Makes 4 drinks.

QUICK MORNING SMOOTHIE

2 Frozen Bananas

1 cup of sliced frozen peaches

1 cup of natural apple juice

½ cup of sliced strawberries

Place all ingredients in blender, mix and drink

ROOTIE TOOTIE BANANA SMOOTHIE

Fruit Drink
½ sandwich bag frozen bananas
1-2 cups any other fruit you have handy, frozen or not
1 small tub yogurt
milk if needed
ice
Put about 1 ½ cups ice into a blender. Blend until pieces are about 1/3 inch across at biggest. Add yogurt and blend a bit more. Add bananas and other fruit slowly, a couple pieces at a time, and blend in between adding them. Add more ice, or add milk if needed to adjust consistency.

SAINT SMOOTHIE

3 nectarines, peeled and de-stoned
2 bananas, sliced
1 cup nonfat vanilla yogurt
crushed ice
2 Tbsp grenadine

Place the nectarines and bananas into a blender along with the yogurt and whisk it all together until it has a good consistency. Next, fill the glasses a quarter with crushed ice, and pour over the grenadine. Top the glass up the rest of the way with the smoothie mixture, and enjoy. Serves 2

SOUTHWEST SMOOTHIE

1/2 c Banana; sliced

1/2 c Mango OR papaya OR guava (Fruit should be of one kind listed and be chopped)

2 c Milk

1 tb Honey

Place all ingredients in food processor workbowl fitted with steel blade or in blender container; cover and process on high speed until smooth. Strain if using mango. Serves 3.

SPARKLING FRUIT SMOOTHIE

1 c Yogurt, plain or -fruit-flavored

2 c Chopped fresh fruit

Freshly grated nutmeg - pinch

2/3 c Ice-cold champagne, -sparkling water or ginger -ale

Mint sprigs (opt) -OR Fruit slices (opt) -(for garnish)

Combine the yogurt, fruit, and nutmeg in a blender; process until smooth. Pour into glasses, filling 3/4 full. Top off with champagne, sparkling water or ginger ale. Gently stir to combine. Garnish with mint sprigs or fruit slices, if desired. Serves 2.

STRAWBERRY SMOOTHIE

5 large strawberries

6 oz. light (reduced sugar) fat-free strawberry frozen yogurt (This is one container of Yoplait)

4 oz. Crystal Light or other sugar-free lemonade

1 packet Equal sweetener or 2 teaspoons of sugar (1 gram)

Put all ingredients into blender. Blend until smoothie consistency is reached! Serves 1.

STRAWBERRY BANANA SMOOTHIE

1 cup frozen strawberries

1 cup frozen banana cubes

1 cup pineapple juice -- or more if needed

2 tablespoons cream of coconut

1 dash grenadine garnish: ripe strawberries

Combine all ingredients in a blender until smooth. Add more pineapple juice if needed. Serve immediately. Yield: 2 servings

STRAWBERRY BANANA SUPREME SMOOTHIE

1 cup strawberry nectar or apple juice

1 cup milk
1 frozen banana
1 1/2 cups frozen strawberries
1 cup strawberry yogurt Pour all liquid ingredients into the blender. Add all frozen ingredients. Blend at MIX setting for 30 seconds then blend at SMOOTH setting until smooth. While the machine is running, move the stir stick around counter-clockwise to aid mixing. Serve immediately. Each recipe serves 3-5.

STRAWBERRY-BANANA TOFU SMOOTHIE

½ cup apple juice
½ cup frozen vanilla nonfat yogurt, peach sorbet, or desired flavor sorbet
4 ounces (1/2 cup) soft tofu, drained
1 cup fresh or frozen sliced strawberries or peaches
1 banana, broken into chunks
1 teaspoon honey
½ cup ice cubes
Fresh whole berries for garnish (optional)
1. Place the apple juice, sorbet, tofu, strawberries or peaches, banana and honey in a blender. Cover and process until well blended. 2. With blender still running, drop ice cubes, one at a time, through the hole in the lid until smooth. 3. Pour into tall glasses; garnish with a fresh berries, if desired. Makes 2 -3 servings

STRAWBERRY FRUIT FROST SMOOTHIE

1 1/2 c Strawberries, stemmed

2 Small or 1 1/2 large Bananas, thorougly ripe Broken into 1 inch pieces

1 c Frozen or canned peach Slices

1 c Apple juice

1 tb Honey

1 c Ice cubes

In blender container, combine all ingredients except ice cubes. Blend until smooth. Add Ice cubes. Blend until smooth Serves 2.

STRAWBERRY LEMON ZING SMOOTHIE

2 cups lemonade
2 cups frozen strawberries
1 cup strawberry yogurt Pour all liquid ingredients into the blender. Add all frozen ingredients. Blend at MIX setting for 30 seconds then blend at SMOOTH setting until smooth. While the machine is running, move the stir stick around counter-clockwise to aid mixing. Serve immediately. Each recipe serves 3-5.

STRAWEBERRY PEACH SMOOTHIE

1 cup strawberries or more
2/3 cup peach yogurt
3 tablespoons of sugar
1 cup ice

Blend all ingredients together until smooth!

STRAWBERRY PEACH & PEAR SMOOTHIE

1 peach, stoned and sliced
1 pear, peeled, cored and chopped
200g (7oz) strawberries, frozen and slightly thawed
good squeeze of lime

Put everything into a food blender and whiz until smooth. Serves 2.

STRAWBERRY PINEAPPLE SMOOTHIE

3/4 bag frozen unsweetened whole strawberries

4 cups Dole pineapple juice

1 cup orange juice (fresh-squeezed or Tropicana Pure Premium recommended)

1 1/2 cups lowfat vanilla yogurt, frozen

Put all ingredients into blender. Blend well, stopping to stir when necessary, until smoothie consistency is reached!

STRAWBERRY SOY SMOOTHIE

1 cup vanilla soy milk

5 ounces silken tofu, firm, chilled and cubed

2 cups frozen or fresh strawberries

2 tablespoons honey

1/2 teaspoon vanilla

Combine in blender. Makes 2 shakes.

STRAWBERRY ZEST SMOOTHIE

10 oz Frozen sliced strawberries -- thawed

4 c Milk

1 pt Strawberry ice cream

1 tsp Lemon rind -- grated

Combine all, one half at a time in blender on high, 1 min. (Or use a mixer). Serve in tall glasses. Serves 8.

SUNSHINE SMOOTHIE

1 cup orange sherbet (or substitute frozen yogurt)
1 cup fresh strawberries, trimmed
1 1/3 cups pineapple chunks, fresh or canned in juice and drained
1 1/2 cups sparkling mineral water

Blend first 3 ingredients in a food processor until smooth; add mineral water until blended.

Serves 4

SWEET STRAWBERRY SMOOTHIE

1 strawberry/mango yogurt (any kind will do)
1 cup fresh strawberries, cut up (or you can use any kind of fruit that's in the yogurt you desire)
½ cup of sugar
1 cup chopped ice cubes
Combine the strawberries (or any kind of fruit) and sugar in the blender and mix on second speed into a liquid. Add the yogurt and blend until mixed thoroughly. Add the ice a little at a time until it's completely mixed. Enjoy!

TANGERINE BERRY SMOOTHIE

½ cup lowfat or nonfat plain yogurt
½ cup tangerine juice
½ cup frozen, unsweetened strawberries, unthawed
1 tablespoon sugar, or to taste
In a blender whirl all ingredients together 30 seconds to 1 minute until smooth and frothy. Makes 1 serving; about 1 - ½ cups.

TANGY SUMMER BLEND SMOOTHIE

1 nectarine

6 oz. light (reduced sugar) fat-free peach frozen yogurt (This is one container of Yoplait)

1/2 c. Dole Pine-Orange-Guava juice

1/2 c. Crystal Light or other sugar-free lemonade

1 packet Equal sweetener or 2 teaspoons of sugar -- (1 gram)

Put all ingredients into blender. Blend until smoothie consistency is reached! Serves 1.

TRIPLE FRUIT SMOOTHIE

1 banana
4 slices fresh or frozen peaches
4 fresh or frozen strawberries
10 ounces apple juice or cider
1/8 teaspoon cinnamon

Place all ingredients in blender. Blend until SMOOTH! Pour into chilled glass and garnish with fruit and a dash of cinnamon. Serves 2.

TROPICAL FIVE FRUIT BLAST SMOOTHIE

1 large banana, peeled and cut into 1-inch pieces
2 kiwi fruit, peeled and quartered
1/2 cup peeled and diced mango
1/2 cup peeled and diced papaya
1 cup freshly squeezed orange juice
3 ice cubes

Combine all ingredients in blender and whip until smooth. Serves 2

TROPICAL PARADISE SMOOTHIE

1 1/2 cups pineapple-orange juice
1 cup sliced banana (about 1 medium)
1 cup ice cubes
3/4 cup diced pineapple
1/2 cup vanilla fat-free frozen yogurt
1 tablespoon flaked sweetened coconut
Combine all ingredients in a blender, and process until smooth. Serve immediately.

TROPICAL PASSION SMOOTHIE

1 papaya
1 peach
2 passionfruit
150ml (5fl oz) freshly squeezed orange juice

Method Peel the papaya and remove the seeds, put the flesh into a blender. Wash the peach, halve, remove the stone and chop the flesh, then add. Halve the passionfruit and scoop the seeds straight into the blender with the orange juice. Blend. Serve poured over ice with the remaining passionfruit on top. Serves 2

TROPICAL SMOOTHIE

2 1/2 cups pineapple juice -- unsweetened

1 cup strawberries -- sliced

1 banana -- sliced OR mango -- diced OR papaya -- diced * If using mangos or papaya, make sure they are ripe.

Peel and dice the fruit. Have the pineapple juice well-chilled. Combine all ingredients in a blender. Puree until thick and very smooth. Serves 4.

TROPICAL TOFU BERRY SMOOTHIE

I cup light (reduced sugar) fat-free vanilla yogurt

1 cup skim milk

1 banana

3" cube of soft tofu

3/4 cup blueberries

1 cup strawberries

Put yogurt, milk, banana, tofu, and Equal into blender and blend until smooth. Add berries and blend again until smoothie consistency is reached.

TUTTI FRUITY SMOOTHIE

1 cup sliced ripe banana (about 1 medium)
1 cup orange juice
3/4 cup sliced peeled peaches
3/4 cup sliced strawberries
1 tablespoon honey
Combine all ingredients in a blender; process until smooth. Serve immediately.

TWICE BERRY BANANA SMOOTHIE

1/2 ~ 1 cup yogurt
1/2 ~ 1 banana
1/2 ~ 1 cup blueberries (fresh or frozen)
1/2 ~ 1 cup strawberries (fresh or frozen)
Juice from one orange (when in a bind I have used orange juice from a carton) honey or sugar to taste.
Mix in blender till smooth.

WAKE & SHAKE SMOOTHIE

3/4 cup orange juice
3/4 cup nonfat yogurt
1/2 of a medium papaya (peeled, seeds removed)
1 teaspoon lime juice
1/2 banana
3-4 ice cubes

Place all ingredients in a blender. Blend until smooth! Serves 1.

WILD BERRY FREEZE SMOOTHIE

1 cup orange juice
1/4 cup pineapple juice
2 pineapple slices
6 fresh strawberries
15 frozen raspberries
10 frozen blackberries
15 frozen blueberries
3 oz. favorite berry yogurt (optional)
ice cubes

Place all ingredients in a blender; blend until SMOOTH. Pour into chilled glass and serve.

YOGURT SMOOTHIE

1 Banana

1 1/2 cup Dannon Vanilla Yogurt (fat free)

3/4 cup frozen peaches

1 whole frozen strawberry container

1 tablespoon orange juice concentrate

Place all ingredients in blender, add ice to fill blender and blend. Serves 2.

YOGURT FRUIT SMOOTHIE

In Blender Add:
2 C Vanilla Yogurt (or fruit flavor)(I like Old Home brand)
1 Banana - cut up*
4-5 Strawberries*
½ tsp Vanilla or Almond Extract
1 Tbsp Sugar or Equal
Enough Ice Cubes to fill blender loosely
Sometimes I freeze fresh strawberries and cut back on the ice. You can add more or less of any of the ingredients. *You can use whatever type of fresh fruit you like, approximately 1-1/2 - 2 C worth.

YOGURT SHAKE SMOOTHIE

Yield: 2 Servings
1 C Plain yogurt
1 Small Banana
1 T Frozen orange juice
Sugar or honey, to taste
4 Ice cubes

Yields about 2 l/2 cups. Place all ingredients into blender or food processor. Whirl until smooth. Variations: Instead of banana, use l cup cubed melon, l/2 cup fresh or frozen berries, l/2 cup pineapple, l peeled and chopped kiwifruit or l/2 peeled and cored apple.

www.ingramcontent.com/pod-product-compliance
Lightning Source LLC
Chambersburg PA
CBHW041512280526
45792CB00004B/1231